THE LITTLE SCHIZOAFFECTIVE BOOK

by
Mark Freeman BSc

CONTENT

- An overview
- Symptoms and Types
- Diagnosis
- Treatment
- Self-care and Self-Management
- Nutrition and mental health
- Alcohol
- Exercise
- Accepting the Condition
- Mindfulness
- Thank you

This book is intended for anyone outside of a clinical setting, who wants a simple explanation of what schizoaffective disorder is and what it is all about, coping strategies and self-management. From those recently diagnosed, experiencing symptoms or those who care for someone who experiences this disorder or perhaps someone who has an inquisitive nature and a few hours to spare.

AN OVERVIEW

First let's start with the basics, and an understanding of what this mental health condition is, I will from now on refer to it as a 'condition' and not a 'disorder' as horrific and scary as this condition can be, I often find as a diagnosed Schizoaffective myself, that a healthy way to frame it, is as a condition, much like asthma is a condition.

It is merely a set of collective symptoms that find their way to the surface of one's behaviour, that needs regulation and management. That's all it is, yes, it is very complex, and no diagnosed person is like the one before or the one ahead, each person is an individual and so, as such is the presentation of the condition.

Schizoaffective, is a condition that affects around 1 in 200 individuals, in a town such as where I live there are statistically a few hundred living amongst me, and they come in all shapes and sizes, ethnic background, gender, age, employment, social level, rich and poor.

The condition cares not about one's car, bank balance, age, marital status, weight, height, political alliances, religion or colour. Even if you deny its existence, it will not care about that either. Every website will present you with the same information, it is a condition of two other mental health disorders Bipolar and Schizophrenia, and in my experience, I will say that is accurate, but in some respects it can be vague.

Researching this condition, one is suddenly presented with

two other complex and separate mental health disorders (Bipolar & Schizophrenia) to get to grips with, so bipolar you may think is straight forward, but alas it is not.

Remember we are delving into a human brain, after all, there is nothing in the known universe that is as complex as a human brain, so be proud that you are the lucky recipient of one, even if it at times feels like burden. Then having looked on bipolar websites and books you emerge with glazed eyes to look up about Schizophrenia, again another incredibly complex disorder too. I suspect after that one shuts the laptop down and has a cup of tea or a paracetamol like I did eight years ago.

Now let's look at bipolar, there are a few types, no doubt if you are diagnosed and in treatment for the conditions, this may feel like I'm trying to teach you to suck eggs but bear with me. Bipolar 1,2, mixed and cyclothymia, are all mood disorders under the ever-expanding bipolar umbrella.

One can expect to and experience at least one episode of Mania, Hypomania, depression and those at the severe end of the spectrum hallucinations and delusions. But, wait, isn't that Schizoaffective? I hear you ask, well yes and no, like I said, conditions are complex and Schizoaffective kind of has its feet on both sides.

Schizophrenia is a its core a thought disorder, it translates in Latin as splitting of the mind, and is in all likelihood the most misunderstood and misrepresented disorder in mental health, in media from films to newspapers the schizophrenic has been portrayed as a psychopathic killer without reason or cognition, to a multiple personality maniac incapable of navigating his or hers daily life.

Now earlier I said **I** and not **We**, well as such is the strength of the myth that Schizophrenia is a multiple personality disorder, that everyone who I have ever disclosed that side of the condition to has quired about which person I am today or have I ever hurt anyone. The answer to those questions is simple, 'me' and 'only myself'.

So, in effect you my friend have a 'thought' 'Schizo' and 'Mood' 'Affective' condition, sounds basic, in fact if one was to say 'hey

I have a thought condition' the other person may respond with a blunt 'eh?' equally if you were to say 'I have a mood condition' you would probably receive a similar confused response, and that's natural, after all mental health is still misunderstood for the most part amongst the general public.

But what does it mean, really, well the diagnosis is merely a 'tag' or a 'label' so that a clinician can refer to the ICD-10 or the DSM 5 (Manuals used by clinicians for a diagnosis) for information about your diagnosis if they need as such. They are likely to find the following symptoms

- Depression
- Mania or Hypomania
- Hallucinations
- Delusions
- Unusual thought patterns
- Catatonia

And so on, those few symptoms bring so much with each one, depression is a killer, mania can derail relationships and employments, hallucinations can cause great distress, delusions will do everything it can to keep you away from reality and catatonia will render one a statue. Once told that you the financial wizard, the pro gamer, the nurse, the bartender, the primary school teacher, the naval officer, the customer service advisor, the cook, the bin man, the writer and so on are victim to a disorder, it can be quite difficult to grasp. Now you sir or madam, display a set of symptoms that will crush you and marginalise you, derail your life to such an extent that you can lose it all and may never get it back. Very scary and that's how I felt, in fact getting a diagnosis back then triggered a severe depression. But I'm here to say if you've just been diagnosed please fret not, you will carve out a successful and fulfilling life, just like you deserve.

But you may only experience a few symptoms, not many suffer all, some do, even then with right treatment they can function. That's all treatment aims to do, is help one back to a normality, back to work or to a functionality that doesn't require enhanced care, but such is the condition not all unfortunately achieve that and that's the reality of mental health.

SYMPTOMS & TYPES

Now when addressing symptoms, one must consider the individuality of the condition, as mentioned very few suffer all listed symptoms and some only get a few. They are however as follows.

The Schizo 'Thought' part of the condition is the Schizophrenia aspect so one can experience symptoms such as

- Hallucinations
- Delusions
- Catatonia
- Disorganised speech
- Disorganised behaviour
- Negative symptoms

Yes, quite a menu of a mental mess, yet when broken down and explained much easier to digest.

So first off **Hallucinations,** in simple terms this means one will see and experience things that do not exist. These can be visual (seeing things) or auditory (nearing things i.e. voices) my hallucinations are very specific and in no way related to the environment, for example, I will see 'The Shadow Man' from time to time, or I will 'Hear The old Lady' or general overlapping whispers and voices both male and female, amusingly I was once in conversation with a woman who was in love with me and said I was fabulous albeit it was all in my head.

I've met those who don't have visual hallucinations but do hear voices, I met someone who is so inundated with voices that he has great difficulty in following simple instruction and much worse from individuals in psychiatric wards that I won't go into.

Each are unique and vary, but all can be disturbing. Also hallucinations can be tactile to mean that one might 'feel' things on them or around them that simply are not there, they can be olfactory in nature that is you may smell something that isn't there, some have even been known to call the fire bigrade as they smelt an thick burning smell, even food can taste completely different, I myself have been subject to that, I've bit into fresh apples only to spit them out in disgust as they tasted like bile.

Delusions again are unique but still disturbing and causes destress for the sufferer and family and friends, you may seem 'lost' to those who love you, and by all accounts you are. My delusions have ranged from government conspiracies to murder me, to the police framing me, then only to be convinced I'm going to prison, I'm been recorded or poisoned. Another type can be that you are a person of great ability and importance, I've known those who believe they are a millionaire, even when checking their bank account they will twist around the facts to only confirm their wealth, I've heard of people on benefits walk into an estate agent to buy a six bedroom house or walk into a BMW dealership brandishing a bank card and demanding a test drive of their latest sports car. Or the usual outburst of self-importance, and 'Don't you know who I am?' Additionally, a common delusion of mine is when TV or songs are a point of reference, I will at times believe that TV hosts are talking directly to me, I've heard coded messages in songs and newspapers.

Some people believe that their thoughts are been transmitted over the world, again, I want to impress on you that the delusion may be very different each time, but the damage it can cause is unpredictable so treatment at the earliest opportunity must be sought in all breakthrough symptoms no matter how inconsequential they may appear to be.

Catatonia is not something that I've personally experienced, I have met others who have, and they all say in a roundabout way one thing, they feel stuck in a moment, I think we all have moments, albeit very brief where we just zone out and stare off into the distance. I'm guessing its clinical form of that, but little is known about this type of symptom those who do suffer from it also switch to been very active to inactive and even silence.

Disorganised speech is as it says, one's words and sentences have no flow, or appropriate reference, you may assume you are making sense, but to those around you its pure gobbledegook! Trust in them when they tell you that, it's also identified as 'word salad' there no connection or link to anything your saying. You may talk quickly or to slow, jumping from subject to subject without even a word to bridge them. I do this very often; I know when I'm doing it sometimes yet if I don't catch it early enough, I will talk a length at anyone near me of every jumbled sentence that happens to pop into my mind. I even joke about it (strange I know) my friends have said they can't follow me sometimes, and some of them make a point of how it must be scary not to know my next thought, to which I ask my friend 'Do you know *your* next thought?'

Disorganised behaviour again, will be behaviours that are typically not what you would do, you may dress different, skip meals, not eat, not wash, spend hours fixating on a subject or topic, go to places that you wouldn't usually and engage in behaviour that is out of sorts.

Negative symptoms can range from, lack of movement, no sex drive, no motivation, great difficulty in planning, reduction in speech, drastic change in sleep patterns, poor hygiene, you may feel emotionless and not look people in the eye. You'll be hard pressed not find a Schizoaffective or Schizophrenic that does not experience negative symptoms.

Such is the nature of these symptoms that they are very hard to treat and have a just as an impact if not a greater impact than the positive symptoms (Hallucinations, Delusions etc) as they last far longer.

As well as these come the cognitive issues, which I see more as by-product of the chaos and confusion that the main symptoms bring, so you may have a poor memory, or have trouble storing information in your brain, you may not be able to follow complex instruction, I have trouble often following recipe instructions, yet I love to cook, which is frustrating.

Also, you may not be able to pay attention to things, I sometimes hesitate to watch a new TV show in case I lose track of the plot. The impact on daily life is almost limitless, you can navigate it, and manage in such a way that one can function to the point that the condition isn't obvious to others even people you work with or friends.

It's worth keeping in mind that recovery is common in the U.K 3 in 10 people have a long-lasting recovery and at least 1 in 5 have significant improvement. That's not to say that you will fully or never recover from an episode that contains Schizophrenic symptoms, but it's worth noting all the same, treatment can and does work, and recovery is not an impossibility, far from it. So that is the Schizo side the part of the condition that's concerned with thought and behaviour of course behaviour can mean anything really, it's all about context and meaning.

◆ ◆ ◆

Moving on to Bipolar, on the surface of things bipolar seems like a relative stroll in the park, even fun! But it is far from it. I even go as far as to say that most reactions to when I told someone I was bipolar were positive, 'oh cool' or 'you must be a painter' or 'yeah like Stephen Fry, he's great!' all left me smiling back polity in disbelief.

Bipolar can be very damaging, can end relationships and crash your car, empty your bank account and give you an alcohol addiction, it can plant you in lifestyle that you can simply not maintain. Bipolar will write cheques for thousands of pounds to charities and it will walk you onto oncoming traffic, yeah how cool is that! Not very!

Before I was diagnosed Schizoaffective, I was treated as having Bipolar 2 even sent to bipolar support groups, needless to say I felt somewhat out of place in these groups, some I could relate to but not all, as coming across a voice hearer was not that common, some did.

As I mentioned earlier there are a few types of bipolar, so there is type one and type two, the main difference between them is the type of mania associated with them, type one has typical Mania, that is a prolonged period of time in which you will have increased energy, decreased sleep if at all and over activity, you will be most likely unstoppable in your goals and may even be incredibly social even charming.

Hypomania is associated with type 2, this translates as 'below-mania' and is shorter lasting and less destructive, some I've met some who have called it 'a buzz'.

Mania can last weeks or months and be very destructive money seems to be at the core of it for many, as it fuels and funds the lifestyle that they engage in. For example, someone who is manic will be full of ideas, very talkative somewhat like the disorganised speech in Schizophrenia but with a direction and end goal. Plans pile up on each other, their thoughts will be whizzing around at hundreds of miles an hour, they will have very far reaching goals that normally they would feel impossible. But now it's easy, they can learn new tasks better, drink more, do drugs, smoke more, exercise more, not sleep and shop, and shop a lot.

My mania has directed me to the bank to withdraw all my student loan money and head into town, I would call friends and invite them to a pub where we would spend 12 hours or more drinking and eating, I would gamble, I would smoke, I would drink pint after pint and then run off to a shop to try and buy a new TV only to run back midway through a sales transaction, much to the annoyance of the sales assistant.

Back then my behaviour to most seemed generous, confident and fun. I would talk to women all day and even get numbers, now that is a complete change for me, ask my friends I'm terrible with women! Yet when manic I'm a regular lothario, of course that's what I think and I'm in fact waving money at them saying do you want a drink? Drunk people are very suggestable to more drink.

The internet has made shopping so much more accessible, I can look back to my late teens when manic and becoming very angry that the high street was closed, in my twenty's I sat with glee as I went on eBay and Amazon, the smile soon wiped from my face when the rent was due.

That's a brief personal account of mania, and just one of many, such is the nature of Bipolar it is episodic, so one will have episodes of increased activity and excess only to trail off into normality but sooner or later that crash will come, and one will suffer from a depression that is very hard to shift.

Some people have longer highs and more intense, some have months after of just plodding along nicely then they are hit with a low mood to depressed, some suffer more than others with the depression, again it's all different for each individual. Knowing the early warnings signs can reduce the severity of an episode, also of course medication does help greatly, but I will get to that later.

The third type of bipolar is called cyclothymia, and is episodic too, only a sufferer will have very frequent episodes, its reported that one diagnosed with this type will only be symptom free for two or three months a year, however they never suffer full blown mania, it will be Hypomania which only lasts days and then cycle into depression and then to hypomania.

Many with cyclothymia can develop Bipolar one or Two, again mood is fluid, so it stands to reason that the disorders are to.

Another type is mixed type where someone may have mania and depression at the same time (or shift between the two very quickly they will be low in mood but be full of energy and restless, a very strange feeling and quite alarming. There are rapid cyclers where a sufferer will have over four depressive and manic episodes in year.

Looking at the manic symptoms its worth listing the main symptoms of mania, that is the ones that a clinician will look for in assessment, they are;

- Full of ideas and plans
- Feeling elated
- Very talkative
- Unable to sleep
- Overconfident
- Taking much more on than you can handle
- Bouncing from idea to idea
- Making life changing decisions on an impulse
- Miss management of money
- Engage in damaging behaviour such as excessive alcohol or drug use, promiscuity, gambling, spending money you don't have to spare

So that can manifest in several ways, but in simple terms you want to live like a Rockstar! However, you probably don't have the bank balance to back it up.

Now we narrow to our condition a pick n mix of the two, a little mania here sprinkled with hallucinations and a dollop of depression, all very disturbing and with ability to turn one's life upside down and leave a trail of destruction in its wake.

So, the three types are Schizoaffective mixed type and Schizoaffective depressed type, both fair self-explanatory, mixed simply implies the mood or 'affective' part involves both Mania or Hypomania and Depression with the Schizo 'Thought' side.

The 'Depressive' type, again self-explanatory, one does not experience any elation or mania, only depressive episodes and there is 'Manic' type only mania is experienced and not depression. Either way, both are not pleasant, even Hypomania can be very disruptive, one might feel great and full of ideas, but they can quickly become very irritable and confrontational.

DIAGNOSIS

I think it is appropriate to highlight here how a diagnosis is achieved, as I know that Dr Google can lead individuals to a self-diagnosis, which is a very dangerous thing to do, it may be that you suspect that you may have this condition.

There are many online tests, that while seem to have the relevant questions needed to diagnose, they are very misleading and vague, I have filled in online tests just to see and some of the questions are too broad to give any real insight.

For example 'Do you hear voices' well of course, but so do lots of people, nearly all have heard a voice a few times, typically calling their name, or in the middle of the night, one will be more likely to hallucinate these hallucinations are known as Hypnagogic hallucinations.

If one was to answer questions on hallucinations, well one's answer would be yes, now you're 50% to a diagnosis on google. Add a few questions about excessive behaviour and mood, well you can see how one can get carried away.

Only a qualified mental health professional diagnoses you and trust me it will likely take a while before they do, it took me three years under psychiatric care before I was accurately diagnosed. As mentioned, I had a working diagnosis of bipolar type 2 with thought problems prior to my Schizoaffective diagnosis.

Now one may feel that a trip to the GP will end in a diagnosis, well it won't a GP cannot do this, they lack the in depth knowledge to do that, mental health conditions are so varied and complex that even when a GP treats depression they will perhaps throw pills and CBT at you, beyond that one needs a consultant psychiatrist.

The reasons why one needs a specialist aside from the obvious is that they can provide a treatment plan that is tailored and effective, they have quicker access to a variety of medications (GP's cannot provide a first prescription of Mood stabilisers and antipsychotics etc).

Consultant psychiatrists are primarily the one to diagnose you, I've always seen them as the key holder to the cupboard of treatments, they can assess you far more accurately than Dr Google. Having assessed, they unlock the cupboard if needed and start to pick out an initial treatment. It must be noted that treatment is at first a trial and error process, as there are many treatments available, a consultant will try out various combinations to see what is effective and what is not.

Specifically, what criteria must be met to be diagnosed Schizoaffective, first of the symptoms must be at disorder level, so the voices, shifts in mood, mania, hallucinations or delusions and so on, must have a significant impact in your ability to function appropriately, and have a significant impact in one's ability to perform daily tasks.

If one is so depressed that they can't wash or eat well it's safe to say, then that said depression is of a clinical nature etc. The episodes one experience must be of a length of time too, Mania must be from my experiences of speaking to psychiatrists longer than seven days, although I've known those who have shorter times with it, but it's not that common. Hypomania must be at least four days. Depression some say at least two weeks, and as far as the Schizophrenic side goes some consultants may wait a year before they consider factoring that in as a disorder. That to me on paper at first glance sounds unfair, I had to go about eight continues months of hallucinations and voices etc, before I was diagnosed, that is not to say I wasn't treated for it, as soon as I mentioned that I was hallucinating again and hearing things, I was immediately subscribed an antipsychotic, and rightly so, even with the absence of a Schizoaffective or Schizophrenia diagnosis.

The internet may be a good starting point, so if you have recently started experiencing symptoms associated with this condition or any other mental health disorder, however, please do not assume that an online test is accurate. Some of these tests only exist to pump up pharmaceutical companies' revenues. I've seen tests run by pharmaceutical companies and filled them out incredibly conservatively and at least come out with a suspected bipolar condition and I must seek a consultant. I cannot stress enough, again please take the online stuff as superficial, only an accurate diagnosis can come from a consultant psychiatrist. So do some research and then go to your GP who can refer you, this process can take a couple of months.

If one requires urgent care, then and I hate to say this the police are the most accessible route to removing one from a situation that might be causing harm to someone or yourself. They can at least provide a safer environment, however they are in not experts, one can expect them to try and find a bed in ward for you or a relative that can care, it's not entirely a done deal that police intervention will help but it's an option.

The idea really is to get in the system, to have it documented that one is experiencing disturbances, once you are in the mental health system then it is far easier to access treatment, even if it's ever without consent (sectioned). As stretched as the mental health system can be it is full of wonderful, empathetic and well-trained dedicated staff who can provide not just care but an outlet for emotional support also.

What to do if you have now decided to visit the GP, well first of reward yourself for the recognition that something isn't right, let me assure you, you are not crazy! Yes, technically you may be unwell, after all mental illnesses are real and are illnesses.

Once you have booked the GP appointment, what is needed to prepare, now you may just think that when you're sat in front of the GP you can just start reeling off symptom after symptom and the GP will instantly treat you.

Well, not quite, they can if they feel the need to send you to urgent care, a phone call to a psychiatric ward may be one option, but if you're able to book an appointment I'd guess that you are perhaps in a fairly Compos mentis state.

You have a few minutes to convey the last weeks or months to the GP, it is best I find, to write down the symptoms that you have experienced, or have a friend or family member do it, as often those are the people who can highlight behaviour that is not typical for you.

Once written take that with you and relate best you can that you for an X amount of time have been experiencing symptoms, explain that it is having a significant impact on your daily functions and tasks. You may have been off work as a result, or unable to study at university or if unemployed you may find that you are not sticking to one's typical routine and having problems with daily activities.

There are many ways this condition will manifest itself, and particularly if it's your first experience articulating the chaos may be difficult without help. If you feel comfortable take a person you trust with you ideally who knows you very well. They can describe your behaviour to a GP if you are unable too, so with written information and a person there to help you with the GP, one stands a good chance of been sent in the right direction.

The GP may not provide treatment at this point, one reason for this is that if you have had mania a GP will be hesitant in prescribing antidepressants particularly SSRI's as some people with bipolar will become manic on them, for some reason antidepressants interact with a bipolar brain to the point where rather than levelling out ones mood it raises so high that the mood spills over the threshold required for mania.

After the GP (if you don't require an early intervention team at this moment) you will have to wait to see a consultant. This is a strange time, on my first referral I had to wait three months before I saw a consultant psychiatrist, some may have to wait less some more.

During this time, I was lucky that my symptoms somewhat decreased in severity and I could navigate my days more effectively, not as I could when I'm well, but I managed. Now you may be waiting and feeling like you are getting worse, again go back to the GP, call the police, even walk into A&E do whatever you can to get back into the system.

The urge to self-medicate with drugs and alcohol is hard to resist but please be aware that self-medication is ineffective and will only make things worse. I understand that some have self-medicated for years, but ask them has it worked and the answer will be no, I have not met a diagnosed schizoaffective person who said drugs or alcohol worked in the long term, in fact these substances reduce your ability to handle the symptoms and at worst will bring on new a more severe set.

Now you are ready to visit the consultant, this can be scary, all of a sudden it may become official, I am the only person in my circle of friends and family that had ever been sent to a consultant psychiatrist, that was enough to bring the hammer of reality down on me at the time.

I even considered cancelling, and to this day I thank my lovely brain that I didn't. Please do attend, even if you feel that this was all not that bad, maybe you feel you were just stressed and tired, please just go even if it's just to eliminate a mental health condition as a cause. They will ask a broad variety of questions, delving back many years if need be, from their initial assessment if needed they can prescribe appropriate medication and so begins the treatment process, and the first steps into recovery. A blood test may be requested too, sometimes bipolar symptoms can be as a result of an underlying physical condition i.e. an overactive thyroid.

You should at this point congratulate yourself on seeking help, you are a brave person with courage to face a difficult process. Yes, treatment is at first difficult, I will come to why later. Again, as with the GP document your symptoms, and if possible, bring a friend or family member who you trust and knows you well, even if it's just for emotional support.

Now in the system, please keep openminded and engage with treatment, they will find the right combination for you, it may take a while, but it will happen. If you need a reference as to where they get the diagnostic criteria from they typically come from the ICD-10 or the DSM-5, you can google these books, they are the bible of mental health conditions and go to for all mental health diagnosis and conditions. I mention this as I want to assure you that a diagnosis is not a person's best guess or opinion, you must meet criteria to be diagnosed.

TREATMENT

Having been diagnosed it is likely that you are now been treated, initially you can expect to be on medication. For mixed type you will be prescribed a Mood stabiliser and antipsychotics, possibly with antidepressants although in my experience the addition of an antidepressant is as a result of a recent depressive episode.

If you do have mixed type an SSRI will likely be withheld until needed. With Depressive type expect to on antipsychotic and a SSRI (antidepressants) and finally with Manic type it will be sometimes just a mood stabiliser but usually an antipsychotic will be introduced accordingly. There are many types of Antipsychotics, mood stabilisers and antidepressants and it may take a while to find the right combination for you, remember the brain is very complex so it will react differently to each medication.

One must get the balance right, its somewhat scientific but really the adjustment of medication will all likely depend on your experiences of them, a more accurate account of the effectiveness and side effects from you will help in finding the right medications. I feel it is worth noting that even on medication one can still become unwell, pills are not a cure, they do work, but life is subtle and unpredictable.

Not to say that medication is not worth it, far from it, after years of been on medications I can confidently say that my life has significantly improved, but one has to engage with treatment too, such as therapy and lifestyle changes, one simply cannot expect to neck a pill and then go back to a unchecked lifestyle, you may have change diet, reduce alcohol etc but I will come to that later.

As well as the above medication types, you may from time to time be prescribed meds that are designed to slow you down, what that means is a sleeping pill might be needed in the interim, or a strong anti-anxiety medication such as Xanax or clonazepam, they all are addictive, so do not expect to be on these for a long time, most likely you will get no more than two weeks' worth. It is best to develop an affective and natural self-management plan in respect to the condition, yes easier said than done I know.

The more you can build up your resistance to anxiety for example the less need for addictive medication, been addicted to Xanax is like having another disorder to deal with, the idea is engage in treatment but not be 100% dependant on the NHS a lot of it will come from you and your family and friends. It must be noted that there are charities that provide support and you can find local support groups that do not need a referral, that's worth a google, I have found groups and charities to be incredibly effective and I consider them to be a great source of treatment, so do look for them (some listed at the end of the book) I'd even go as far to say they should be integrated (especially support and social groups) into your treatment plan.

Medications come with the dreaded side effects, yes, they are sometimes just as bad as the symptoms they are designed to treat, the information sheet of each medication is an unsettling read. You now find that you possibly will have to manage a whole host of side effects as well as the symptoms. That's why at first it is a difficult process to treat such a condition, these meds are powerful, they are designed to target very specific chemicals that are involved in more than just mood or thoughts. For example, mood stabilisers and antipsychotics target the dopamine system, dopamine is a chemical in the brain that is involved in mood, feeling happy, addictions, rewards and even the fluidity of body movement. So, when staring on these medications you may feel restlessness (known as akathisia, there are pills to treat that if it becomes unbearable) your arms may not move smoothly, walking may be a little difficult and so on. Here is a list of there more common experiences, some are far worse and may even result in person hospitalised, although this is rare. More common are;

- Dry mouth
- Drooling
- Restlessness (akathisia)
- Shaking hands
- Weight gain
- Drowsiness
- Stomach aches
- Tremors
- Nausea
- Feeling dizzy
- Vomiting

After reading that one might want to not take them, people are afraid of the side effects or becoming a zombie like figure remaining motionless on the sofa, and I completely understand that, nobody really wants to be a shaking vomiting dizzy person who gains weight. It's not a nice feeling and can make it feel that it's not worth the trouble.

I will admit my first weeks on medications was horrible, I cried, I drooled, I shook, I was sick, I hated it, but after a while the side effects for the most part ware off, the body is incredible in that it can build up a tolerance to the medication.

Once the side effects are now not a problem, you start to evaluate along with the mental health team the efficiency of the prescription, the aim really is to eventually get to a stage where the symptoms are significantly reduced while at the same time you can still function as normally as possible. There is no use in have a dosage that eliminates all symptoms but the side effects prevent you from carrying on with day to day activities, in all likelihood you will continue to have breakthrough symptoms from time to time but as long as the quality of life is there, one can begin to integrate self-care and self-management into the treatment plan.

SELF-CARE AND SELF-MANAGEMENT

I feel that this requires a whole chapter dedicated to it, this maybe the most useful chapter for you, here I will provide coping strategies and self-treatment of this condition, not all will work for you, and you may have some not listed but hopefully you will find some to try out in here.

I will start with self-treatment of the Schizo side of the coin then move onto the affective part, again, there is no guarantee, these techniques will not eliminate symptoms but will give you a way to cope with them while in treatment and on medication.

First let me impress on you the importance of acceptance, one can spend a lifetime trying to accept this condition, but once you do, life becomes easier, you will still have the symptoms and episodes but you will fell a more complete person by framing this condition as much as a part of you as your organs or fingers etc. It may not define you, but you do have it and as it is chronic and no cure is on the table, it will be lifelong and always there, yet with treatment and self-management you can lead a very rich and productive life, even using your condition and experience to effective use, so keep that in mind.

Voices, so annoying, exhausting, distracting, scary, horrific and even amusing at times, yes amusing like I said sometimes my voices are funny even complementary, but that's very rare and hasn't happened for years, typically they are mean and nasty to put it crudely.

I will not repeat what they have said in the past. So personally, my go to coping technique is an obvious and simple one, most likely it may be what you do. I get my iPhone I plug in my headphones and listen to music to drown them out, been a guitar player myself I sometimes plug my headphones into my guitar amp and play my guitar. But first I try the music through headphones, now this is assuming that you are on medication so this is more of a breakthrough of a positive symptom which will happen.

Some like to listen to their favourite artists some even download tinnitus apps which I do too (I have tinnitus) these apps have great distraction noises that you can train the mind to zero in and focus only on, then I find the voices while still there, just feel further away.

Reading can be a good distraction too when the voices or hallucinations are not to severe, particularly if you try to read from right to left, this gives the brain something to concentrate on rather than the hallucinations.

Exercise too can be incorporated with music, so sometimes when I hear voices I put my headphones on and I do sit ups or I follow a low intensity home exercise YouTube video, again this gives you a way of distancing yourself from the hallucinations, they may still be there after you finish but you might feel more space between you and them.

Meditation, is a counter intuitive way to deal with hallucinations, I stumbled across this technique while trying to manage my tinnitus, I was meditating and then I started hearing voices, which were distressing but, given the relaxed state I was in I found the strength to continue mediating, after a few minutes I found that the voices had quietened, they were still saying the same things but I could hardly hear them, so I continued meditating. It was unexpected and as far as I'm aware not a recognised coping technique, it is counterintuitive to sit in silence while hearing voices. So if you are thinking meditation, two things are essential, one you have to learn the skill of meditation, it is a very effective way of clearing and calming the mind but it is not learnt overnight, it took me around 6 weeks to really get decent enough at it, but once I acquired the skill it was an essential part of self-care, it is if used right a workhorse of self-care, it works well with anxiety, confidence, sleep and much more. Secondly practice mediation every day, even twice a day if you can, 15-20 minutes at a time and typically you will build up a resistance to your triggers and symptoms and reduce the distress of the condition.

Sometimes the simple act of ignoring them can help, often if situation will not allow for headphones etc I simply ignore them, it's not easy or ideal, some people can complete ignore them, I do this by shifting my focus elsewhere, so if you're in a public situation, take in the surroundings, the sounds, the people, the smells, the colours and so on, I would even create back stories for people I'd see, or count how many dogs on walk or my steps, find whatever works for you, it's not a difficult as it may seem.

Singing is a good distraction, I am a terrible singer but that doesn't stop me, I sing and I sing proudly when I have to, put on a cd and sing away, pick an engaging song with a upbeat positive vibe, for me it's queen 'don't stop me now' is my go to song, so much fun to bounce around too!

Painting is a great distraction too, find a nice spot outside (weather permitting) and paint the scene, or indoors make a little corner in a room dedicated to creative pursuits, don't limit yourself be ability or lack of, the end product is not important, it's the process.

Phone a friend! Yes, so simple but effective, you can choose to tell them why you're calling, up to you, but find a subject that you love to talk about and put the word to rights.

A quick run round the block, I have a dog so if experiencing hallucinations, we go for a run, he enjoys it and I ger a healthy distraction, plus the adrenaline boost helps, and the release of positive chemicals flood your brain. The link between exercise and mental wellbeing is well documented, the rule should be to exercise every day, do what you can, don't overstretch yourself as inactivity and injury can trigger symptoms. So, you may find an app or a DVD to exercise daily. Your body and mind will be very grateful.

Respond to hallucinations in a rational way, answer them, tell them they are wrong, even go as far to dedicate a five or ten minute window where they can have their moment, then move on, in doing this you are practicing acceptance, you letting the voices or hallucinations know, that you acknowledge them but they have no influence, that is a very powerful message to install.

While paying attention to hallucinations remember that one, they are not real and two, they only in your head, no one else around you are involved. Look for evidence to contradict them, tell it to go bother someone else and you're not scared, because it's from your brain so let them know that without you they would not be here, you can dismiss them.

Another technique I use, is to write down all the things in life I'm thankful for, all my achievements, my favourite things etc... or I write a short story, writing is a great distraction it engages creativity and concentration, both a very good combination. A colouring in book also can draw your attention away, I have an adult swearword colouring in book, very amusing it is too. A warm bath can be used although I personally have not benefited from this, but some swear by it, make the bath a safe zone, put relaxing music on, bath salts and relaxing oils and aromas, allow the senses to enjoy a relaxing environment.

If you are really struggling phone the local crisis team, they are available out of hours and can help, it is even sometimes calling them just so they can email a nurse or psychiatrist to call you the next working day.

Coping with the 'Affective' side is a different ball game, in the same sport but different rules, I personally find that the coping strategies are less about distraction and more about reducing the impact of an episode.

Mania, as mentioned is very destructive and disturbing, so it is essential that you have a crisis plan set up, you can personalise plan with friends and the mental health professionals treating you. I will say that it is very helpful to have someone know what your triggers are and how mania or hypomania presents itself.

First it is very helpful to get to know your moods, not many people do this, some simply get happy and accept it as that, anger is just anger and a bad mood is just that and so on, but moods differ in intensity. So it's worth learning what a genuine and situation appropriate mood response is for you, the best way to do this is to track your overall daily mood, this is best done at the end of the day, sit down for a few minutes and assess where you are, some score on a scale 1 to 10 but I find using the 'plus 5, minus 5' scale better, minus 5 would be major depression and plus 5 would be elation or mania, 0 would be natural. If you are an excel whizz you can track moods on there and come up with a line graph, there are apps to that can help some are better than others, over time you will start to see a pattern. It is also worth noting the events of the day that have driven your mood a bit lower or higher, so you can start to identify triggers.

Learn your early warning signs, so many overlook the very early stages of mania, yet they can be vital, if left unchecked one can become ill, if nipped in the bud you may prevent an episode. Some may find early signs such as obsessing about shopping and an urge to buy, or some may start talking a bit more or faster, some may start planning more or getting less sleep, even feeling bit more irritable. Whatever they may be it is best to address them quickly, they may or may not be a start of an episode but there's no harm in seeking a little help or self-care, get that extra hour in bed back if you can, distract yourself from wanted to buy things, go exercise, you will find thigs that work for you eventually.

Stick to a routine, it is very important that you have a routine and structure in your life, ask anyone who just watches TV all day how the feel, most likely not good. Employment provides a good structure but not all can do that, part time employment might be better along with a hobby or other interests. Take time if you can in the day to practice mediation or mindfulness, and a relaxation hour. Also make cleaning the house or flat a daily task, I love cleaning it practices focus, give you a little exercise and a clean house just feels better, do not underestimate the environment in which live in, a untidy place will affect you more than you realise. Here is my typical routine for my day

Morning take my dog to the garden to toilet, prepare breakfast, take morning medication, one coffee, one banana, one apple and one slice of toast. Feed my dog. Shower, brush teeth and put on deodorant. Put on some music and tidy my flat. Hoover, polish, dust, make/change bedding, clean all rooms until satisfied. Rest, 20 minutes watch TV or play a game on my computer. Walk dog. Relax. Then in 30-45 minutes of indoor exercise. Wash again. Relax.

Afternoon, eat lunch, meditation for 20 – 30 minutes, read for a while, write down anything that I need to do later or tomorrow, watch a bit of TV, engage in a creative activity. Play with my dog. Try and learn something new.

Evening, make dinner, walk the dog, play a game with dog, feed him, take evening medication and supplements, mediate for 10 minutes, read for 30 minutes, watch a new TV show or a favourite, listen to music.

Obviously that's a rough day in my life, life is subtle and fluid, ever changing, things crop up, so remember that while a routine is essential, allow yourself so wiggle room, a mental health nurse who runs very effective support groups said 'It's like driving a car with one foot riding the break' and I agree, one has accept that if you are to engage in unhealthy behaviours and lifestyles then you will have a harder time coping.

Now that looks like a non-eventful day, and to some extent they are, but that is what we ideally want to have, a run of the mill somewhat structured day, you may be in full time work, or have children or both. That's great because they are obviously your

structure, been an employee and all that comes with it is structure, raising children is structure. But taking time out when you can to engage in creativity or relaxation is very effective at providing that self-worth and enjoyment that well all need regardless of mental health diagnosis. A day with purpose is very good, even if today's purpose is cracking on with the very mundane run of the mill things that we all do, shopping, school run, reading, cooking, cleaning etc its far better, cheaper and less stressful than mania. But understand that if stress is now a major thing in your life, then you will need to act, stress is a huge weight, it lowers the immune system and is linked to mental health problems, over time it can be very serious. So, take time to stop, breath and step back from things, as best you can.

Managing finances is so important, engage in budget planning, crisis planning and intrust a trustworthy person to act as probate. At the start of this chapter I advised on a crisis plan, and you should make one if you already haven't. First you need to recognise the early warning signs, so a colour system of 'GREEN, YELLOW and RED' is the simplest way to see if intervention or a medical review is needed. Discuss with loved ones and medical professionals about putting a plan together. Also write down, what you feel is a light episode that is you may only have a few symptoms that are not to disturbing.

This would most likely be in the 'GREEN' zone, so a few symptoms enough of note but not destructive. Once you've consulted with the crisis plan, then you can or others decide what's best, perhaps a small increase in medication or an earlier appointment.

If you're symptoms are serve and you are in the 'YELLOW' or 'RED' zones, then that may involve an assessment, if extremely severe and you feel unsafe hospital admission may be needed. It is all down to how your life is affected, no one knows better than you, so if you feel that recently things have become a little wobbly, then go look at the plan, what zone if at all are you in?. This will give you hopefully a sense of control. On the zones you can include not only symptoms, but 'observable' behaviours, friends and family members will also pick up on any unusual speech or activity. Below is an example of a 'GREEN to YELLOW' list and what to do,

GREEN ZONE (slightly unwell) – Symptoms and observable behaviours.
- Reduced sleep
- Spending money
- More interest in alcohol
- Over talkative
- Some peripheral hallucinations
- Hearing voices
- Excessive talking
- Checking of locks to much
- Looking out of the window for any sign of intruders

Treatment plan: Call community mental health team for advice, possible assessment for increased care, medical review, others to document behaviour, engage with mental health team, ring crisis team if needed, hand over bank card to trusted person.

YELLOW, (quite unwell) Symptoms and Observable behaviour
- Sleeping 2-3 hours per night
- Quick to anger
- Irritable
- Hallucinations
- Voices (cruel and threatening)
- Paranoia
- Checking locks on doors and windows
- Spending too much money
- Obsessive behaviours
- Excessive drinking/drug taking
- TV talks to you

Treatment plan: Assessment under the mental health act if needed. Increase home visits from mental health nurse. Medical review. Call crisis if out of hours. Possible prescription of a strong antianxiety medication and/or sleeping tablet. Review after three-four days. Partner to keep an eye for more behaviours.

As you can see in this very general crisis plan, there is a system set up ready to jump in and slow everything down for you, I find during these times distress that the world is too quick, my mind is too busy, it's all chaos and soon enough I will lose my grip and ability to function.

The involvement of others is needed at these stages, they will document assess and treat you as needed. If left unchecked and one slips in a RED zone, then that's a bad and unpredictable place to be in as you many know. You will have noticed that the GREEN and YELLOW symptoms are similar in parts, this is because that as you may know you can have a severe symptom such as hearing voices but nothing else, symptoms can overlap into different zones, so keep track of what you are experiencing refer to the colour charts and see what place you are in.

I feel in doing this it gives a sense of power over the condition, while you may be having symptoms, having recognised it and classified it by the severity, you or a friend or family member can start to act, take back what the condition is trying to take from you, and step away in a safe controlled manner.

We just focused on the manic and though problem side of things, but depression and anxiety are all too common if you are Schizoaffective, even if only diagnosed manic type we all get down days and it's possible to develop depression even if you have never experienced it. You may find the following tips on preventing a relapse and recognising an approaching depressive episode, as is with mania and hypomania prevention is far better. Learn as with manic episodes the triggers and early warning signs, engage with treatment of depression and educate yourself about the condition.

Common signs of a depressive episode are subtle and may seem unnoteworthy yet again like mania if left unchecked you can sleepwalk into an unpleasant situation and much worse. It's all about the preservation of health and to that end one should learn and implement.

So, you may start to crave junk food or chocolate, sleep patterns change, feel like withdrawing from people, avoid doing the things you typically enjoy, and skip meals. You may also start having physical symptoms such as head and back aches, stomach issues or changes in bowel movements.

While a crisis plan is a very useful tool if you have started to become or are now unwell. A wellness kit as it where is great in keeping a lid on the symptoms and giving you a platform to build on, also this kit is packed with the things you enjoy and activities which reduce stress and anxiety.

The kit may look something like this;

- A good night's sleep on a regular basis
- A reduction in activities, not taking on more than you can handle
- Attendance of a local support group
- Check in with a person you trust and is supportive
- A call to a GP
- Engage in creativity, paint, draw, play an instrument, write etc
- Practice relaxation, deep bath or sit and simply watch the world pass you by
- Keep your house or flat sunny! Have the windows open if its nice weather allow light to fill your world
- Seek some help with tasks if you feel overwhelmed
- Reduce caffeine, alcohol, nicotine and sugar
- Increase stimulation or if need decrease

Another good thing to do is reach out to new people or engage with people in your life more, Schizoaffective individuals, at times like Bipolar and Schizophrenics can isolate themselves.

I in the past would begin to withdraw from my friends and family and not once has it worked out well.

Of course, time alone can be very helpful, it's a subtle condition, withdrawing from the outside world can allow one to reflect and plan, gather one's thoughts and contemplate on what next. But isolation is entirely different, it will hinder recovery and limit your coping strategies, at these times it is helpful to have a loved one check in with you every day, a phone call or a visit for a chat and a cup of tea. If however you are the type of person who naturally withdraws even when feeling well, then it would be a good idea to drop a message to a trusting person and a mental health professional (if you are in care) to advise them of the situation, and check in with them frequently. Again, complete isolation is never advised, so keep in mind that e around you care, so let them support you. If you are at the stage where delusional behaviour and thoughts is the overriding symptom/s then it may be appropriate for professional intervention, even a stay in hospital, in any case if you are in a severe state then this may well happen with or without your consent. You may not be in a place to recognise how unwell you are, but behaviours do not go unnoticed and help will arrive.

NUTRITION AND MENTAL HEALTH

Now we all know the mantra "you are what you eat" and it's one that I've always agreed with but not until the last few years understood. The link between food and mental health is an obvious yet understated link. How often will a GP tell you exercise more if your depressed? Or lose weight, like they are the magic cures.

Life is not that black and white, and neither is nutrition. As this is a disorder of the brain, it only stands to reason that we treat it carefully and give it the proper nutrition it needs. We do the same for our heart, liver and stomach, yet how much consideration do people give to their brain? At a push some will eat fish once a week because they've heard of Omega 3 fatty acid, beyond that can many name other food sources for a healthy functioning brain.

Yet it is vital, not only to emotional wellbeing, cognitive function, decision making, sleep, memory but also in prevention of mental health issues, and even in aiding recovery. What is remarkable that much more research goes into advertising junk food, chocolate and alcohol, than ever goes into researching mental health nutrition, and in all my years of mental health care and intervention never have I had a meaningful discussion about diet. I'm sure there are access to this form of treatment, but it must be rare.

We all know "an apple a day keeps the doctor away" well yes and no, apples are healthy, but one cannot simply buy seven apples, one a day and have an unhealthy diet surrounding it, it just will not work out well. So, what are the recommendations then, what food should one be eating? The key is to not make your diet feel like a chore, otherwise you will not eat well, and it's not about removing enjoyment, or stopping the occasional cake or even a beer from time to time. In fact, drastically reinventing one's diet will most likely cause stress and lead to you abandoning it all together. Remember the tale of the tortoise and hare? Who wins the race? Exactly. So, if food is something that you need to change then do it gradually, start by swapping out items.

But this is not a diet book, what we need to keep in mind when food shopping, is what vitamins and ingredients are going to promote health? Well there are a number, we already know of Omega 3, that is a good start, so swap out a burger for a healthy portion of fish, salmon fried in olive oil with backed potato and a cheeky spice is far better for you. It may not light up the reward centre in your brain, but over time it will be very happy about that fish dinner twice a week. Vegetables are the base on which your meals should be built on, every meal I have I immediately think vegetables the recommendation (in the U.K is five fruit and vegetables a day), what goes well with which one. I know, boring right? Wrong! Invest in a vegetarian cook book, and add things you like (as long as they are good for you) I take inspiration from a vegan book, I add fish or sometimes chicken and it works a treat, also with the activity of preparing a tasty, well balanced and healthy meal, only adds to wellbeing and a sense of achievement (that's why there's so much money in good food, people want to eat it, dine out on it, cook it, read about it and watch tv about it! How many of us want to watch a KFC kitchen or McDonalds worker flip a burger?). Get creative, treat cooking the same as any hobby you enjoy, always look to try new healthy foods without prejudice, remember how rubbish you feel after a takeaway? Sure, at first all that sugar and fat sends your brain into a little high, but your body feels no such effect, and long term it only leads to poor physical and mental health. Keep in mind a well-balanced diet with plenty of fruit, veg and water will help more than you can ever know (if you don't already have a balanced diet) and remember no one person ever regrets eating healthy food.

If you have no clue as what nutrients are good for you here is a few and what foods contain them;

- Vitamins B1, B3 and B5, *found in wholegrains and vegetables, these help with depression, concentration, attention, stress and memory*
- Vitamins B6, *found in wholegrains and bananas, help with irritability, memory, depression and stress*
- Vitamin B12, *found in many sources of meat, fish, eggs and dairy products, helps with memory, psychosis and confusion*
- Zinc, *found in Nuts, seeds and Fish, helps with confusion, blank mind, depression, motivation and appetite*
- Vitamin C, *found in vegetables and fresh fruit, helps with depression*
- Selenium, *found in Fish, garlic, sunflower seeds, Brazil nuts and Wholegrains*
- Folic acid, *found in Green Leafy vegetables, helps with anxiety, depression and psychosis*
- Magnesium, *found in Green vegetables, nuts and seeds, helps with insomnia, depression and irritability*

You can see from just introducing more fruit, fish, nuts, seeds and greens onto the plate each day you can build up a resistance to a whole host of mental health issues, so the benefits are there to be had, as well as keeping the body healthy, you will find that this will have a positive impact in other areas of your life.

It is also worth noting that many studies have successfully found a link between processed foods, high sugar content, additives and saturated fats and poor mental health. Even individuals with a serious mental health condition are frequently found to have a poor diet.

ALCOHOL

We all like a drink from time to time, a nice cool pint on hot summers day with friends, what more can you want? So appealing isn't it, we British love a drink, we are a nation of drinkers, every weekend the cities are awash with booze! Even the romans would remark about our affinity with wine.

But alcohol and mental health have a strange and complex relationship, too much of it too often, can lead to depression and then when depressed one drinks even more. Alcohol first and foremost is a depressive, it's not an enhancer, it's not an upper, at first you will feel a slight euphoric feeling or relaxed, but after a few more drinks that can swiftly change into a low mood and even aggression.

It interferes with sleep patterns, which is a big red flag for a schizoaffective, no sleep will only lead to trouble. Is the buzz worth the lack of rest? Probably not. Short term it may help with difficult situations or a stressful time, but as long as you recognise it as an occasional thing and have a healthy relationship with alcohol then it can be part of a balanced diet just look at the Mediterranean diet red wine is included, although rule of thumb I'd look to cut it out entirely and save up for a holiday!

If you are using alcohol to self-medicate and many do, I myself did at first, you need to understand that alcoholism or alcohol used as a medication will only reduce your ability to lead a productive life. You will sleep less, eat bad foods, have more mood problems, arguments, engage in impulsive depending sprees, poor decisions and even be more violent. Alcohol is a toxic substance, it affects areas of the brain in ways that are problematic, that first drink might give you a relaxed feeling, but sure enough as more enters the blood stream, your inhibitions are lowered, movement will be affected, emotions are magnified making you prone to switch mood states at the most inconspicuous of reasons, and sexual desire increases but sexual performance decreases, that's probably why most one night stands are a huge let down!

The other problem with alcohol is that you build up a resistance to it, it takes more to get the relaxed feeling or if any mild euphoria, so you drink more to cope with anxiety and depression, but the more you drink the less effect it has and the more it adds to your anxiety and depression. As it depresses the central nervous system and has an inhabiting affect. This amplifies our feelings making you feel worse. It's a self-perpetuation that only serves to harm you, it is best if you can to avoid alcohol as a medication, same said for drugs and food.

Many studies into the effects of alcohol on mood shown that while most reported a relaxed feeling, very few reported feeling less anxious, socially comfortable, less depressed, more confident, able make friends and feel in control. Most people drink to relax, which is fine, but if you drink to 'forget' or fell less anxious, the short of it, it just won't work, just ask any alcoholic how their drinking to cope worked out. It's surprising really that alcohol consumption and misuse is very common. As with food try and remember moderation is key, ask why you are drinking, to what end? And do you enjoy been drunk? I myself do not drink any more, I was never a big drinker anyway, so I found it easy to cut out the drink, and I can say I've never felt better for it.

EXERCISE

I touched briefly on exercise and the benefits it brings, all of us know the link and it is well documented that exercise has multiple health benefits. Improving mental and physical health, you may think that to exercise you need an expensive pair of running shoes or a gym membership, well you don't. There are many ways to exercise, a lot can be done in your living room, all you need is accessed to YouTube or a DVD player. Pop on an exercise routine video that suits you. The government recommends thirty minutes a day, to some that sounds a lot but there are very achievable ways to hit that target by simply doing things a little differently. For example, if you normally drive to the supermarket for the weekly shop, try walking to a local shop or high street to pick up part of the shop, walk to work etc, keep active, walk round the block a few times a day. You will find that once you work in exercise into you daily routine your mental health will improve, it will (just like a healthy diet) have a positive impact in other areas of your life that you didn't anticipate.

Studies have shown that people report more positive feelings after a short period of physical activity than after non activity, feeling calmer, more content and more awake. Even after a period of low mood a short time exercising had an immediate increase in mood, with people reporting that after a walk or brief exercise they felt happier than thirty minutes before where they felt a little low. Many studies have even shown that walking 30-35 minutes a day 3-5 days a week over 10-12 weeks improved mood, enthusiasm, reduced stress, increased alertness and improved wellbeing of those with a serious mental health condition. There is even evidence that suggests that exercise withdrawal has a serious effect on mood, with people reporting that removing an exercise routine from their day left them feeling down, more depressed and more anxious. There is a wealth of evidence about the subject, it is highly advisable that you take part in physical activity on a daily basis at least 3 times a week, there is no down side to exercise if done right, even if you just walk thirty minutes a day you feel the benefits.

ACCEPTING THE CONDITION

It can be tough to live with a Schizoaffective diagnosis, when I was first diagnosed my heart sank, I was awash with images of future conversations with friends, family and colleagues, and yes, I was too concerned about the stigma I may face. Not many know about the condition, and most have a negative association with the word Schizo, so receiving a diagnosis can bruise you. But, there is no getting away from it, to be honest the term Schizoaffective on really exists for the clinicians, so they can tick a box or input a DSM code into the system, or when you see a new doctor they know what symptoms you experience. It could be called anything, if it was called green shoe disease it would still be the same set of symptoms and require the same treatment, what is in a name after all?

It is vital to accept the condition, if you don't accept it then how can those around you? You will find that once you do, living with it will be easier. What does acceptance mean? It doesn't mean liking the condition or enjoying it, or even choosing it. But if you push back against it or try to reject it you only create an internal struggle with it, you create another layer of pain, an allowance for the condition will help you get space from it. By giving yourself permission to be Schizoaffective, to be who you are, what you feel, what you experience, you may not rid yourself of displeasing experiences, but you will elevate some of the pain associated with them.

Acceptance will not happen overnight, like any new skill it takes practice, it is natural at first to feel resistance to the diagnosis, but make space for accepting it, over time it will become something that you live with, engage with and accept. It doesn't mine that you are your condition, far from it. A person with asthma would say they are asthma or someone with diabetes wouldn't say they are diabetes, so would you say 'I'm Schizoaffective', I don't, yes I have Schizoaffective but that's just one part of me, I also have tinnitus, a bad back and a perky attitude!

But I am not defined by my conditions, they have all influenced my outlook on life and in ways my personality, to ignore the impact and influence the condition has is to deny it. Which naturally we know will make you feel worse, I accept that sometimes the condition and I (as a person) overlap and lines blur, but equally the line is well defined, I can say when I feel paranoid for no reason that that's not me it's the condition, then I can start to distance myself from the paranoia. Be kind to yourself, if you find that you are allowing low mood, or paranoia for example to exist then don't beat yourself up for it, try just noting it 'Oh, I feel a bit anxious' 'Oh I just saw something' and then move on, note and move.

Acceptance is not giving up and just living with it in pain, it's not apathy, quite the opposite, practising acceptance allows you to make positive changes in your life, you may find that accepting this condition that other areas of your life will improve and even you may feel more comfortable in your own skin. Also it doesn't mean that because you do accept the condition that it will be like this for ever, the one thing constant in life is change, and mental health is no different, many people who engage with acceptance, a healthier lifestyle, exercise, reduce drugs and alcohol and engage with treatment recover and even experience fewer relapses.

MINDFULNESS

Now I will finish about practicing mindfulness, it almost sounds like hippy approach and a bit counter intuitive, naturally the condition presents scary thoughts and feelings, so been mindful of them is the last thing you may want to do. But practising this will help you get some head space away from the unpleasant experiences. It is worth noting that mindfulness while been proven to be very helpful in depression, worry and anxiety, there is little evidence in the way of treating psychosis.

What is mindfulness? At its core it is routed in Buddhism and mediation, what it asks you to do is try to be present in the mind and body, without judgment. In practising mindfulness, over time you will be able to become more self-aware, cope with difficult thoughts, be kinder to yourself and reduce stress as well as allowing you to choose how you respond to unhelpful thoughts.

There are few ways to develop this skill and they are simple to do; all require you to be present in the moment. Mindful eating is a great way to start, when eating a meal pay special attention to the taste, texture and smells of the food, is it spicy? Is it sweet? How nice is it? How salty? Also note the space around you while you eat or drink, how does the fork feel in your hand or cup of coffee? Note the feeling of sitting and your feet on the floor, the feeling of the air on your skin. Mindful drawing can be a great way to develop the skill further, pay attention to the detail, the colours, the sound the pencil or brush makes as it draws on the paper, there are mindfulness colouring books available so investigate that.

Body scan is also a helpful technique, this is where you scan your body by moving your attention slowly down from the top of the head to the edges of your feet, note the feelings and sensations you have, warmth, cold, tension and relaxed feelings in the body, don't stop at each one, just scan slowly down and then again for a few minutes at a time.

You can develop the skill as you go about your day, when showering note the water hitting your body and face, try to notice when your mind drifts off and gently bring it back to the now, be curious about feelings and thoughts and not judgemental, and be kind to yourself, don't tell yourself off if your mind does wonder. Finally set aside time to practice take it slowly and be patient, Rome wasn't built in a day.

THANK YOU

So, there you have it, I hope that this little book helped and informed, even if it just confirmed what you already know.

If there was one take home message that I'd like to convey, it would be that life is subtle and fluid, things change, sometimes life is hard and sometimes it is easy, remember you are not your condition, no more than my mother is her bad knee, you are not your unhelpful thoughts, anxiety, psychosis, hallucinations, delusions or depression.

They do not define you.

You should not identify as a schizoaffective, labels are meaningless, nothing more than term for doctors. You are an individual capable of living a meaningful and productive life, we are all individual's mental health condition or not, no two people are the same.

Engage with treatment, try to practice a balanced lifestyle, learn new things, create and develop relationships, keep people in your life who are supportive. Above all recognise when you need to reach out, when things are scary and dark, phone someone, ask for help, go see the GP, been vulnerable is not a weakness, it is a strength.

Love who you are, be kind, honest. Talk about your mental health don't hide it, accept and live your life, do the day to day things that everyone does, don't let the condition stop you. Lastly if things are tough for you right now just know one thing, they will and always do get better in time, but the first step to recovery can only be taken by you.

Thank you for taking the time to read this book

USEFUL WEBSITES AND APPS

Mind.org.uk
Rethink.co.uk
Psychologytoday.com
Verywellmind.com
Headspace.com
Betterhelp.com
Rcpsych.ac.uk
NHS.co.uk
Nice.org.uk
Mentalhealth-uk.org
Time-to-change.org.uk
Sane.org.uk
Youngminds.org.uk
Nimh.nih.gov
Schizophrenia.com
Who.int
Bipolaruk.org
Bphope.com

Dbsalliance.org
Samaritans.org

APPS

BellyBio
Operation Reach Out
eCBT Calm
iSleepeasy
Headspace
Calm
Relax Melodies
Optimism
WhatsMyM3
Sleep trackers
eMoods
Wisdo
ThinkUp Positive Affirmations
The Mindfulness App
Reflectly
5 Minute Home Workouts
BBC Good Food

FAMOUS PEOPLE WITH BIPOLAR AND/ OR SCHIZOPHRENIA

Stephen Fry – Comedian, Actor, TV presenter and Author
Carrie Fisher - Actor
Frank Sinatra - Singer
Mel Gibson - Actor
Charlie Chaplin - Actor
Kurt Cobain – Musician
Catherine Zeta-Jones - Actor
Adam Ant – Singer
Russell Brand – Comedian, Actor and Author
Tom Fletcher – Musician
Graham Greene – Novelist
Terry Hall – Singer
Daniel Johnston – Musician
Chris Kanyon – WWE wrestler
Linda Hamilton - Actor
Jason Nash - YouTuber
Lou Reed – Musician
Rene Russo – Actor/model
Nina Simone – Singer
Ted Turner – Businessman

Jean Claude Van Damme – Actor & Martial arts specialist
Vincent Van Gogh – Impressionist painter
Ruby Wax – TV presenter
Brian Wilson – Musician
Kanye West – Musician
Amy Winehouse – Musician
Bettie Page – Former model
Frances Farmer – Actor
Philip K. Dick – Novelist
Michael Hawkins – Actor
Rufus May – Clinical Psychologist
Elyn Saks – Law professor
Vashishtha Narayan Singh – Mathematician
John Nash – Mathematician and Nobel prize winner
Paul Geosch – Artist &n Architect
Frank Bruno – Boxer
Mariah Carey – Singer
Francis Ford Coppola - Film Director
John Curtain – Former Australian Prime Minister
Larry Flint – Publisher
Paul Gascoigne – Footballer
Phillip Graham – Publisher and Businessman
Teddy Heart – Wrestler
And so many more, you are in good company...

Acknowledgements

I would like to acknowledge and thank my family and friends for enduring my moods and supporting me during difficult times, I wouldn't be the man I am today without their help. A special thanks goes to my Mother, who is the funniest, kind, good hearted and strongest person I know. Thanks for all the support and laughter.

To all those friends, people, colleagues and accountancies over the years, I thank you for all the many interactions that shaped me and made realise that life is full of wonderful (and some not so wonderful) people.

I would also like to thank and acknowledge the amazing and talented NHS staff that have be involved with my mental health treatment at different stages of my life. From been first referred, diagnosed, supported and intervened along my journey. Without them, my recovery would have certainly taken much longer if at all.

Lastly but by no means least, I'd like to thank my rescue dog Winston, for supporting, distracting, never judging and making life fun and interesting, you rescued me.

Made in the USA
Monee, IL
08 August 2020

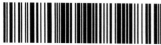

37801062R00035